Alkaline Diet: Raw Food Diet:

Weight Loss for Beginners to Lose Belly Fat & Increase Energy

Emma Rose

Alkaline Diet Guide

Lose Weight Quickly, Achieve Optimal Health, and Feel Energized with the Alkaline Diet and Alkaline Recipes

Emma Rose

Table of Contents

Introduction

I want to thank you and congratulate you for purchasing the book, **"Alkaline Diet Guide**: *Lose Weight Quickly, Achieve Optimal Health and Feel Energized with the Alkaline Diet and Alkaline Recipes"*.

This book contains proven steps and strategies on how you can achieve a more efficient weight loss and at the same time, boost both your energy and health by simply changing the kind of food that you eat. Going Alkaline isn't a new method but for many, the process is still an uncharted road. Let this book be your guide.

Here you'll be provide with an easy to follow process. From start to finish, you'll find all that you need in order to get started as well as enough knowledge to take you to the next phase of the diet itself-- living a healthy, alkaline rich life.

Thanks again for purchasing this book, I hope you enjoy it! Please take some time to stop by and LIKE our Facebook page:

https://www.facebook.com/joypublishing

With gratitude,

Emma Rose

Chapter 1: What Is The Alkaline Diet?

In its basic sense, the alkaline diet (also known under other names such as the acid ash diet, alkaline ash diet and alkaline acid diet) is the belief that certain foods have a significant effect on both the pH and acidity of our body fluids such as blood or urine. With that in mind, it is said that by tweaking these, we can also make use of these food products to help treat certain diseases as well as prevent them. But that's not all-- it has also been said that keeping in line with this diet can also help you lose excess weight.

It's the kind of pitch that anyone would love-- and this is a fact further proven by the Hollywood celebrities who have tried the diet itself. Just take Victoria Beckham for example. But they aren't the only ones who can back up the diet's effectiveness when it comes to weight loss. It all goes back, way back to the time of our hunter-gatherer ancestor's diets.

This is what the Alkaline Diet is based upon, after all. That modern man's everyday diet has basically ruined our metabolic systems (along with other environmental factors), causing it to slow down and become inefficient when it comes to burning up fat from the food we eat. To help you understand that better, here's a quick summary of facts:

1. This "caveman" diet was based on animal foods and minimally (almost none at all) processed plants. However, as time progressed and agriculture became a main source of livelihood for man, the standard Western diet went through an immense change.

2. Grains aren't a typical part of our diet and our bodies, according to the Alkaline Guide, isn't meant to digest these. The same applies to milk, cheese and other derivative products for these were only introduced after the man has learned to domesticate livestock.

3. Sugar and salt consumption rose towards the beginning of the Industrial revolution and in some way, our body never really got used to having too much of it-- way beyond what we can normally get from fruits and other plant food.

4. The diet we all have now is highly acidic and this causes numerous health problems, unsurprisingly. This is what the alkaline diet wishes to change, and basically wants to bring us back to what was more natural for us to consume. Basically resetting our metabolisms-- and making us fat burning "machines" just like our ancestors.

Now, all of that might sound a little complicated but the further we go, the easier it will be to understand. Let's start with acidic food and how it affects our bodies.

Almost all of the food products that we consume, once we have digested and metabolized it, would release either an alkaline base or an acid base into our blood. Grains, meat, shellfish, milk, poultry, cheese and salt all produce acid hence unbalancing the proper pH of our blood (which is slightly alkaline). This kind of diet, if continued and not counteracted by alkaline foods, can cause some serious side effects. Symptoms of a highly acidic diet include:

1. A lack of energy and a sensation of heaviness in your limbs. This can also include a loss of your psychic drive as well as physical tone. You might also feel depressed or an inability to cope.

2. You are more susceptible to different illnesses and infections.

3. You frequently feel cold and your body temperature has significantly lowered. You might also get frequent headaches or dizzy spells.

4. You have dry skin which also tends to experience irritations in areas where you sweat a lot. This is because your sweat has become highly acidic as well and if you have sensitive skin, you might feel slight burning sensations on it.

5. You might also experience stomach pains due to excess gastric acid or acid regurgitation. Ulcers and gastritis are also common symptoms associated with a highly acidic diet.

By switching up the food you regularly eat into something more alkaline, you would be able to avoid all of that and bring back the proper pH balance of your blood. Not to mention the fact that you'll also be helping your metabolism return to normal--making it more efficient when it comes to burning up fat and using it for energy. That alone would hasten the process of weight loss for you.

Chapter 2: Benefits of the Alkaline Diet

Reading the previous chapter might have provided you with an insight as to how the diet works and what it is based upon. However, it does not provide you with any clue as to how it can benefit you-- other than the fact that it would help you lose weight and make your body more efficient when it comes to using the nutrients we get from the food we eat. In this chapter, we'll talk about the benefits and how that affects your overall health.

1. *Improved Energy Levels* – When it comes to your overall level of energy, one of the most important factors would be proper cell function. Basically, if your cells are not healthy then they won't be very effective when it comes to holding as well as transferring oxygen throughout your body. What this results to is fatigue and an absolute lack of energy.

Another factor would be body's pH level. It can significantly affect the cell's ability to provide ATP or adenosine triphosphate, this is also very important to the energy our body is capable of producing. The process of "making" it happens within a cell's mitochondria but if your pH level becomes too acidic, this is hindered. So if you've noticed a recent drop in your energy or if you've been feeling lethargic lately, you might want to look into the diet you've been indulging in. Chances are, the foods you consumed are highly acidic and are messing with the proper pH of your body.

2. *Improved Immune Function* – When your cells are healthy, they are more capable of absorbing the nutrients that your body requires. They are also more efficient when it comes to getting rid of waste products. However, should they be weakened, these functions are compromised as well. As a direct result of this, your immune function is also threatened and you become more susceptible to different infections and different

illnesses. This is among the many ill effects that a highly acidic diet can bring about. Cell damage is just the first of many in the process. So keep your cells healthy by making sure you eat the right stuff.

3. *Slower Aging* – As we have learned, subjecting your cells to highly acidic environment constantly will cause their efficiency to decrease a lot. This also results in its inability to quickly repair itself which leads to premature aging. This happens when the cells don't get enough oxygen and are rendered unable to rid themselves of damaging toxins. An alkaline diet certainly helps in this situation and would help you maintain healthy cells and a youthful appearance as well. Remember that healing your skin doesn't always start from the inside. Sometimes you have to look at the food you eat and make changes to ensure healthy skin.

4. *Reduced Pain and Inflammation* – Magnesium is one of the most important minerals that the body utilizes when it comes to controlling high levels of acid. So if you keep on eating a highly acidic diet, your body would then need to use more magnesium in order to neutralize it. Because of this, it can get depleted thus resulting to tissue and joint pain. Eating alkaline rich foods would help restore the lost magnesium and you'll be able to avoid all of the above without trouble.

5. *Weight Loss* – In changing the food that we eat, we are also able to reset our metabolisms and make it more efficient when it comes to burning food for fuel. The alkaline diet calls for more greens instead of animal protein and that small change alone can help significantly. Remember that our metabolism has a much harder time with animal protein and in time, it actually slows it down. You can fix and clean that up by switching to lighter but no less healthy food products. The same kind our ancestors would have eaten but in proper balance this time. It's all about maintaining that

and making sure that your body is still getting all of the nutrients that it needs to function better.

6. *Healthier Teeth and Gums* – You may not think much about this but a highly acidic diet can certainly affect the health of your gums and teeth. This is because bacteria grows at a much faster rate if your mouth is acidic and that could cause innumerable problems-- starting with bad breath to some serious gum disease. Of course, it also puts you at risk of experiencing tooth decay. An alkaline diet balances even the acids in your mouth so you can avoid experiencing all of that. Many people have noted a significant improvement in their oral health after switching to the diet program.

7. *Neutralizes Acid Imbalance* – An acid imbalance in the body can lead to numerous issues and as such, it should be treated immediately. Just think about the pain that ulcer or hyperacidity can cause. It can be paralyzing in some cases and might even require you to undergo surgeries just so the damage it has caused can be fixed. If you've ever experienced acid reflux then you also know how sick that feels and how much it burns the throat which can also lead to tissue damage as well. Needless to say, this isn't something that you can simply ignore. The best treatment for it isn't medication or surgery-- you don't even need to reach that stage if you simply make dietary and lifestyle changes.

8. *Lowers Risk Factors for Certain Diseases* – It has been said that eating a well-balanced alkaline diet can also help in lowering your risk for developing health problems such as colon cancer and type 2 diabetes. While studies are still being done on it, it's safe to say that the idea isn't too farfetched considering the fact that you'll be switching to healthier foods during the diet and would also need to drop certain bad habits such as smoking if you're to really continue living an alkaline life.

9. *Improve your Heart's Overall Health* – Again, studies are still being done on this but many have said that it did help them improve their cardiovascular health. This is mainly attributed to the fact that the program highly encourages people to eat a well-balanced diet comprised of both greens and meat. It isn't about restricting yourself but instead, it guides you towards finding a plan that works for your needs and that of your health. Cutting back on red meat is one of its core ideas and that alone already helps in preventing certain heart-related issues brought on by high cholesterol.

10. *Detoxification* – Let's talk free radicals and how these things can really take your body for a loop. They are everywhere. In the food that we eat and in our environment so they're not very easy to avoid. Instead, we have to build up a strong defense against them and regularly detoxify our bodies so that they get flushed out long before they have any chance of ruining our cells. However, not a lot of people really pay attention to this and unless they feel something weird happening to their bodies, would still continue on with their bad diet and everyday habits.

If you want to live a longer, healthier life then detoxification is one of the key things you'll need. Eating an alkaline rich diet is one of the biggest steps you can take because it promotes detoxifying food products as part of the meal plans. Couple that with a regular exercise routine and you'll be able to clean up your body in no time. You'll feel its effects almost instantaneously too. More energy, refreshed, brighter skin and eyes, a better ability to concentrate-- those are just a few of the benefits it can provide you with.

Chapter 3: Alkaline Food List

The thing about acidic and alkaline foods is that you can't tell which is which at first glance. Some foods might appear or taste like they could be acidic but are actually alkaline, such is the case of citrus fruits. It is the way our body reacts to a particular food product that ultimately determines whether it's acidic or alkaline.

Now, nearly all vegetable, fruits, nuts, seeds and herbs have alkalizing effects on our bodies though the degrees at which they do tend to vary. Just take tea for example, almost all varieties save for black tea are all alkaline. Rule of thumb is that foods that are not processed and remain closest to their natural state tend to be more alkaline than most. This means that any kind of *processed food such as grains, dairy and fast food tend to be acidic.*

Note that pesticides are actually known to be acid-forming so chose organic when it comes to your fruits and vegetables. Then you have your legumes and beans-- a vegetarian's main source of protein-- which are also acidic. With that said, however, don't eliminate acidic foods from your diet completely. Just make sure that you balance everything well. 60-80% alkaline to 20-40% acidic foods should be just right.

To give you something a bit more specific, here's a quick rundown of the most commonly eaten alkaline foods.

Alkalizing Vegetables

- alfalfa, beet greens, broccoli, barley greens, cabbage, celery, carrot, chard greens, cucumber, dandelions, edible flowers, dulce, fermented veggies, eggplant, green beans, garlic, green peas, lettuce, kohlrabi, kale, mustard greens, mushrooms, parsnips, onions, peas, pumpkins, peppers, nightshade veggies, rutabaga, radishes, spirulina, sea veggies, sprouts, spinach, sweet potatoes, watercress, tomatoes, wild greens and wheat grass.

- dandelion root, daikon, maitake, kombu, reishi, nori, wakame, umeboshi and shitake.

- avocado, apricot, apple, berries, banana, sour cherries, cantaloupe, fresh coconut, currants, figs, dates, grape fruit, grapes, lime, lemon, honeydew melon, nectarine, muskmelons, orange, pineapple, pear, peach, raspberries, raisins, rhubarb, tomato, tangerine, strawberries, umeboshi plum, tropical fruits and watermelon.

- millet, chestnuts, almonds, fermented tofu, fermented tempeh, whey protein powder, stevia (sweetener).

Now, if you're a beginner and have been eating a highly addictive consumerist diet for most of your life then making the switch can be much harder than you think. The foremost reason for this is that your body would eventually crave its usual food and you might end up binge eating because of it too. In order to avoid all of that, pace yourself and start bit by bit. Here are some of the most alkaline forming foods that you can easily work into your everyday meals. Think of them as stepping stones as you slowly transition into a mostly alkaline diet.

1. *Root Vegetables* – Because of the healing nature of these foods, they are often used in traditional Chinese medicine to help with different illnesses. These are rich in vitamins and minerals, more than your average vegetable making it a great addition to any diet. So if you're looking to start simple, try root vegetables as they can also be cooked in different ways. The best bit? They are quite filling so you'll feel satiated after.

2. *Cruciferous Vegetables* – These would include the veggies that many people love. Broccoli, cauliflower and cabbage are just prime examples of this variety. While they are already typically included in your daily diet, you can do more by utilizing them in different ways. As dips or as garnishes, the more you consume of these the better.

3. *Garlic* – When it comes to foods that promote overall health, garlic is among those at the top. It is alkaline-forming but also helps improve heart and immune health. It cleanses the liver and lowers blood pressure while fighting off disease. While it does have a strong smell, there are a number of ways to prepare it which should help with reducing it.

4. *Cayenne Peppers* – This contains enzymes that are actually essential when it comes to our endocrine function-- besides the fact that it is also one of the most alkalizing foods. Not only that, it comes with a rich supply of vitamin A and antibacterial properties which is great if you're looking to detoxify and get rid of free radical in your body.

5. *Lemons* – These are the most alkalizing foods available, and they are also natural disinfectants that are capable of healing wounds. It also energizes the liver and can provide immediate relief if you're experiencing hyperacidity. So a glass of freshly squeezed lemon before or after every meal is a great way of incorporating it into your daily diet. Eating the fruit itself is also great-- if you can stand how sour some of it can be.

Alright, so now that you've got some idea of which foods to pick and which ones you should eat less off, let's move to applying all of it to your daily diet.

Chapter 4: Alkaline Diet Recipes

Let's begin with something easy and quick to prepare for your breakfast. After all, most people would be rushing during this time of day. Using alkaline-forming ingredients, these should provide you with the energy you need for the day.

Spelt Porridge

Ingredients:

- 1 cup of filtered water
- 1/3 cup of flaked spelt
- Powdered stevia or agave for sweetening
- Cinnamon to taste
- 2-3 tablespoons of cranberries or cherries (dried)
- ¼ teaspoon of vanilla

Toppings: hemp nuts, raw nuts, blueberries, hazelnut and hemp milk.

Procedure:

1. Combine your first 6 ingredients and allow it to simmer for at least 3 to 4 minutes before transferring it to a shallow bowl.

2. Once done, sprinkle your toppings all over it.

3. Add your non-dairy milk (almond or hazelnut would work too).

4. Serve warm.

Power Smoothie

Ingredients:

- 1 ¼ of coconut water
- ½ cup of unsweetened almond milk
- A cup of frozen blueberries
- 2/3 cup of frozen raspberries
- 2 tablespoons of agave or stevia
- 1 avocado, sliced
- 3 tablespoons of fresh coconut meat
- ½ a teaspoon of super greens powder
- 4 tablespoons of raw hemp nuts
- 2 tablespoons of omega 3 oil

Procedure:

1. Combine all of your ingredients in a blender.

2. Mince your raspberries and add some more coconut water if you think the consistency needs it.

3. Blend well until it becomes thick and creamy.

4. Yields 4 cups.

Spelt and Vanilla Vegan Pancakes

Ingredients:

- 1 cup of light spelt flour
- 1/8 teaspoon of fine Himalayan salt
- 2 tablespoon of aluminum free baking powder
- 1 cup of almond milk
- 1 tablespoon of maple syrup or stevia
- 1 ½ teaspoon of alcohol free vanilla
- 2 tablespoons of cold pressed sunflower oil
- Coconut oil for greasing

Procedure:

1. Measure all of your dry ingredients in one bowl and the wet ones into a separate one.

2. Give each a stir before combining. Make sure it's mixed well and evenly.

3. Set this aside for at least 5 minutes and allow it to rise.

4. While waiting, prepare your open pan and brush on ¼ teaspoon of coconut oil on it, keeping the heat low.

5. Spoon your batter into this, forming 3 small pancakes. Cook for 3 minutes or until each side become golden.

Hot Chocolate with Coconut Milk

Ingredients:

- ½ cups of unsweetened almond milk
- 10 tablespoons of coconut milk powder
- 1 ½ cup of filtered water
- 6 drops of stevia
- 5 tablespoon of raw cacao powder
- cinnamon
- marshmallows
- 1 ½ tablespoon of agave

Procedure:

1. Using a medium sized sauce pan, mix all of your ingredients together.

2. Make sure you keep the heat on low and whisk until you remove all the lumps.

3. Adjust the sweetness if preferred and serve it topped with marshmallows.

Spring Pea and Edame Bread Spread

Ingredients:

- 1 ½ cup of fresh peas
- 1 ½ cup of edame beans
- ½ teaspoon of salt
- 1/3 cup of extra virgin olive oil + some extra
- 3 stems of fresh mint
- Juice from one lime
- Lime Zest

Procedure:

1. Place your edame beans in boiling water for about 4 minutes until it becomes bright green.

2. Removes them and run the beans under cold water.

3. Repeat the same for your peas except only leave them in for a minute.

4. Once done, place both in a food processor and combine until it gets evenly mixed. Don't puree completely.

5. Add some seasoning and serve in a bowl. A drizzle of olive oil and mint leaf garnish should top it off nicely.

6. Now that you've got easy to prepare recipes for your everyday breakfast, let's talk lunch. Fast foods are definitely part of your options so, what to do? Prepare it beforehand and take it with you!

Raw Zucchini Noodles with Pesto

Ingredients:

- 6 pieces of 8 inch zucchinis, peeled
- 1 cup of basil leaves
- Celtic sea salt
- 3 tablespoons of raw hemp hearts
- ¼ cup of pine nuts or raw cashews
- 1 clove of garlic, crushed
- ¼ cup of olive oil

Procedure:

1. Using your spiral slicer, trim the ends of your zucchini in order to make it line up evenly. Slowly wind it and carefully collect the spaghetti like noodles that would be pushing through the openings on the blade.

2. For fettuccine like noodles, (and if you have no spiral slicer) you can use a simple peeler. Just be careful and mind the thickness.

Pesto Sauce:
1. Combine your olive oil, basil, garlic, nuts and sea salt in a blender. Combine this until you achieve the right consistency. Add more oil if needed.

2. Toss this with your noodles and serve as is to keep noodles nice and crunchy.

Mini Roasted Veggie Skewers with Garlic Basil Dip

Ingredients:

- 1 sweet white onion
- 2 red peppers
- 3 zucchinis
- 3 cloves of crushed garlic
- 12 cherry tomatoes
- ¼ cup of olive oil
- Sea salt
- 12 pieces of skewers

For the dip:
- 2 cloves of garlic
- 1 cup of zucchini
- ½ a cup of extra virgin olive oil
- ½ cup of raw pistachio nuts
- 16 basil leaves
- ½ teaspoon of sea salt

Procedure:

1. Preheat your oven to 400F.

2. Combine our oil and garlic, set this aside.

3. Skewer your veggies, make sure there's a uniform pattern. Set aside.

4. Baste this well with the garlic oil, spreading the garlic bits onto your vegetable pieces.

5. Sprinkle some sea salt over it.

6. Roast for about 15 minutes.

7. For your dip, simply mix all of your dip ingredients in a blender/food processor until it becomes creamy. Add more olive oil if needed.

Now is the time for the good part, which is making healthy dinners. Of course, before bed, you would want something light but no less filling. Try these recipes out and see how it works for you.

Sprouted Grain Wrap with Chipotle Dip

Ingredients:

- 1 peeled parsnip
- 2 medium sized beets
- 1 yellow beet
- 1 large sweet potato
- 4 tablespoons of olive oil
- 1 teaspoon salt
- Mixed greens
- 6 sprouted grain tortilla wraps
- Fresh pea shoots
- Chipotle Dip

Procedure:

1. Toss all of your veggies with oil and salt but keep your red beets separate.

2. Once done, spoon these into your baking sheet, sprinkling the red beets on top. Make sure it's parchment lined.

3. Roast this in a preheated oven (350 degrees) for about 25 minutes until it becomes slightly tender. Remove and allow to cool.

4. Over your wrap pile your greens and spoon some of the roasted roots down its center. Add some of your chipotle dip on top before sprinkling some of the pea shoots.

5. Serve with extra dip and some avocado.

Rainbow Salad with Avocado and Meyer Lemon Dressing

Ingredients:

- Baby spinach and arugula greens
- 1 yellow beet
- 2 carrots
- 6 slices of yellow pepper
- ¼ red onion
- Pea shots
- Micro greens or sprouts
- 1 avocado
- Chopped pistachios

Dressing:
- 1 avocado
- 2 Meyer lemons
- 1 ½ teaspoon of red onion
- 6 fresh dill
- 6 basil leaves
- 1/8 teaspoon of sea salt
- 1/3 cup cold pressed extra virgin olive oil
- 3 drops of stevia

Procedure:

1. Prepare your serving bowls.

2. In each of them place a generous amount of your arugula.

3. Top this with beets and surround that with other veggies. Make sure that everything is layered properly.

4. Add your micro greens, pea shoots and top this with your pistachios.

5. For the dressing, simply process all of the ingredients in a blender. Make sure it reaches a creamy consistency before pouring it in a separate container.

Raw Cranberry Pie to Go

Ingredients:

- 1 organic pear
- 2 cups of raw organic cranberries
- ¼ wedge of orange (keep the skin)
- Juice from half an orange
- ½ cup of raw almonds
- 6 dates
- ½ cup of raw pecans
- ¼ teaspoon of cinnamon
- 1/8 teaspoon allspice
- 1/8 teaspoon ground cloves
- 2 tablespoon of maple syrup
- ½ a teaspoon of vanilla
- 1 cup of untoasted buckwheat

Procedure:

For the base:
1. Soak your buckwheat using filtered water for half an hour. Rinse and drain properly.

2. Combine this with ¼ teaspoon of cinnamon and the orange juice. Add your maple syrup and half a teaspoon of vanilla. Set this aside.

For the filling:
1. Using your food processor, mix your cranberries, your orange, dates, a teaspoon of cinnamon, cloves, all spice and half and teaspoon of vanilla.

2. Make sure this is blended well then set aside.

For the pie topping:

1. Place 2 dates, pecans, almonds and ¼ teaspoon of cinnamon in a food processor.

2. Blend until it becomes crumbly.

3. Now fill your jar layer by layer. Buckwheat bottom, then 2 scoops of the cranberry mixture and topped with the nut crumbles.

4. Top this with some fresh cranberry and seal the lid.

Dairy Free Cherry, Avocado and Coconut Ice Cream

Ingredients:

- 2 cups of cherries + 6 more, finely chopped
- ½ of a large avocado
- 1 400ml organic full fat coconut milk
- 1/3 cup of cashews
- 10 soft dried dates
- Juice of half a lemon
- 2/3 cup of filtered water
- 1/3 cup of cashews, soaked and drained
- 2 tablespoon agave syrup
- 2 tablespoon beet juice (for color)
- Finely chopped dark chocolate

Procedure:

1. Using a high speed blender, combine 2 cups of cherries, avocado, coconut milk, water, cashews, dates and lemon juice.

2. Blend this until it becomes creamy. Taste it for sweetness before adding your agave.

3. Stir your chocolate and chopped cherries into this mixture.

4. Transfer this to your ice cream maker and follow the instructions.

5. You can also choose to freeze this overnight.

6. Garnish with a few more chopped cherries before serving.

So there you have it, some easy to follow recipes that would surely infuse some alkaline into your daily diet. The best bit is that these recipes are actually heart friendly and won't add unwanted calories into your system. If you're trying to lose some weight, they're still perfectly fine to have. Just make note of ingredients that you might be allergic with and switch it to ones that you know are safe for you to eat.

We hope these recipes could serve as the basis for ones that you'll be creating for yourself!

Conclusion

Thank you again for purchasing *"**Alkaline Diet Guide**: Lose Weight Quickly, Achieve Optimal Health and Feel Energized with the Alkaline Diet and Alkaline Recipes"*!

I hope this book was able to help you to better understand how the Alkaline Diet works and how it can significantly benefit you when it comes to losing weight as well as staying healthy and energized.

The next step is to take what you have learned and put it into action. Try the diet and see how it improves your health; find out how it benefits you overall. Keep in mind that the only way you can truly test these things out is not by reading and judging it through that. Putting it to the test and experiencing it is the only way you'll know if it's the right one for you.

Remember, this isn't just a simple diet trend. *It's a lifestyle change for the better!*

Finally, if you enjoyed this book, please take the time to share your thoughts and post a review on Amazon. It'd be greatly appreciated!

In addition, please remember to check out our Facebook page in order to find other resources and upcoming promotions:

https://www.facebook.com/joypublishing

With sincere thanks,

Emma Rose

Preview Of "Paleo Desserts: Satisfy Your Sweet Tooth With Over 100 Quick and Easy Paleo Dessert Recipes and Paleo Baking Recipes"

Introduction

I want to thank you for purchasing the book, *"Paleo Desserts: Satisfy Your Sweet Tooth With Over 100 Quick and Easy Paleo Dessert Recipes and Paleo Baking Recipes"*.

This book contains 100 Paleo dessert and baking recipes on how to prepare delectable desserts without sacrificing your health.

All my life I've had a sweet tooth. I would even go as far as to say that I had a sugar addiction! Over the last few years my sugar addiction got worse: I had dessert multiple times a day and every day (I guess being a Foods teacher didn't help much). I would joke with people by telling them that I had my servings of vegetables for the day in chocolate...except, I still didn't have the vegetables. It got pretty bad. I knew I hated eating that much dessert but I couldn't stop. I would eat one Ferrerro Rocher and then go back for another. As I walked back to the treats, I would pass the mirror and think to myself, "I don't need to have this chocolate. But, ah, what the heck, I don't care." In the end, I'd have about 6 Ferrerro Rochers in addition to the other treats I had earlier that day.

Finally, I had to take the huge tray of Ferrerro Rochers to school to give to my students on Valentine's Day. There was no way I could eat the other 30 myself. Eating all this sugar caused a huge war within me. I knew that my extreme sugar eating was unhealthy for me but I didn't want to stop. I loved it too much. As a result, I wrestled between the ideal of where I wanted to be and the reality of where I was. I knew I had the discipline to say no to other things, so why couldn't I say no to chocolate?

I eventually came to the point where I was starting to get fed up with not feeling well. I had a lot of chronic pain in my neck and I was constantly tired. I knew that sugar was irritating the problem and causing inflammation in my body. At was starting to reach the breaking point. Ultimately, I chose to go off of sugar for at least three weeks to break the habit I had created for myself. It was seriously a miracle to stay consistent with my goal because I really didn't want to give up my favorite desserts.

Shortly after my decision to go off of sugar, I had a miscarriage. Experiencing the loss catapulted me into a massive journey to find health and proper nutrition. I did a live blood analysis with a naturopath to discover what was contributing to the terrible ways I was feeling. Seeing all the garbage I had in my blood forced me to go off of dairy, corn, oats, and wheat. I was left wondering, "What the heck am I going to eat? That stuff is in everything!"

Consequently, I stumbled upon the Paleo diet. It was the most relevant diet to what I was trying to accomplish. I was able to find things to eat for breakfast, lunch and dinner. But desserts were a whole other story. I felt like something was missing and I couldn't put my finger on it. The best I could come up with was apple slices dipped in almond butter: hardly satisfying. Paleo desserts ended up being the by-product of my search to find something, anything that I could enjoy.

I encourage you to make that switch to healthier and happier desserts with the hundred delicious and irresistible recipes presented in this book. You don't need to follow the same extremity that I did. But if you are taking the Paleo diet seriously, then you may find the same void of sweets in your life too. Cutting out all the processed foods and going back to the basics really does clear up the body and help it function better. I've seen the changes in my own life as hard as it's been to make those changes. You, too, can make the changes necessary and still have your sweets along the way!

Thank you again for purchasing this book. I hope you enjoy the recipes. Experiment with them and make substitutions to suit your needs.

With gratitude,

Emma Rose

Chapter 1

Brief History of Paleo Diet

The Sweet Effects

Why do you love sweet food? Why do you crave for more of that dessert so much? Your anatomy would tell you that sweet foods would cause the release of dopamine in the part of the brain that is associated with motivation and reward. Not only that, but studies show that sweets also produce an increased level of serotonin. Serotonin gives you that feeling of happiness and wellbeing. That's why it is better to give a box of chocolates when you want the person to be in a good mood.

Unfortunately, the quote you can't have your cake and eat it too applies here. The bad effects that sugar brings are common knowledge. The number one disease is diabetes. People are aware of diabetes and its complications. That is why even when you intensely crave for that delicious dessert, you try to control your urges and settle for nothing instead. Well, that is if your self-control is in good condition. More often than not, people would rather risk the medical condition and eat that sweet thing with all their heart.

I have had many slip ups in my own life. I went two months without chocolate...can you believe it? Then Easter came. I found that if I gave myself an inch, I would take a mile. Eating chocolate quickly got out of control. I rebelled because I was strict for so long. You may find yourself in the same situation and find it hard to balance the sugar cravings. Once the sugar cravings are there, your body craves more and then a vicious cycle begins.

Check out the rest of "Paleo Desserts: Satisfy Your Sweet Tooth With Over 100 Quick and Easy Paleo Dessert Recipes and Paleo Baking Recipes" on Amazon.

Or go to: http://amzn.to/1lZNcVI

Raw Food Diet Guide

Lose Weight Quickly, Achieve Optimal Health and Feel Energized with the Raw Food Diet and Raw Food Recipes

EMMA ROSE

Table of Contents

Introduction

I want to thank you and congratulate you for purchasing the book, *"**Raw Food Diet Guide**: Lose Weight Quickly, Achieve Optimal Health and Feel Energized with the Raw Food Diet and Raw Food Recipes"*.

This book contains proven steps and strategies on how to effectively apply the raw food diet into your life.

A raw food diet, also known as uncooked diet, is essentially an eating plan that largely involves the consumption of unprocessed and uncooked food. Those who take on this lifestyle are often acknowledged as raw foodists or raw food practitioners. Sometimes, they are referred to as raw food advocates, although this term may also be used to individuals who are interested in or about to convert to the raw food diet.

In the diet, it is believed that cooking or heating of food will destroy the natural enzymes and nutrients typically found in food and produce. This can bring about complications because these enzymes are mainly responsible for fighting off diseases and improving digestion. Therefore, in order to avoid this, raw foodists eat food in its raw state, as the diet's name suggests. This helps alkalize the body, since cooked food has acidic toxins that disrupt the body's acid/alkaline balance. Such disruption often causes illnesses and excess weight. In a nutshell, heating food above 118°F initiates the chemical changes that produce the acidic toxins like free radicals, mutagens and carcinogens, which are normally linked to diseases such as heart problems, arthritis, cancer and diabetes.

There are more than one variations of the diet, and it is entirely up to you how you will shape up your own diet plan. Generally, to be considered a raw foodist, an individual must at least eat 75% to 100% raw, unprocessed and organic food and drink pure water. Most of the items you will eat are plant-based which should never be heated above 115°F. While majority of raw foodists are vegetarian, there are those who opt to consume raw animal products such as raw fish, sashimi, raw milk and the like. Some may also incorporate fresh fruits and vegetables into their meal plan. On the whole, you have the power to create whatever raw food diet structure suits your lifestyle and your preferences best.

Thanks again for purchasing this book, I hope you enjoy it! Please take some time to stop by and LIKE our Facebook page:

https://www.facebook.com/joypublishing

With gratitude,

Emma Rose

Chapter 1

An Overview of the Raw Food Diet

The concept of the raw food diet is simple – cooking diminishes the nutritional value of food. Even though most of the food items in the diet are consumed while it is raw, heating is acceptable provided that the temperature stays between the range of 104 to 118°F or below.

Since cooking is perceived to kill off enzymes naturally found in food, raw food practitioners choose to avoid cooked food. As a matter of fact, overconsumption of cooked food forces the body to work overtime in order to produce more enzymes to support normal bodily functions. In the long run, the lack of enzymes can instigate a lot of problems involving a person's health, particularly accelerated aging, nutrient deficiency, weight gain and digestive problems.

Going raw can prove to be challenging, especially for those that are just starting out. It takes a lot of discipline to stick to the principles of the diet. Moreover, extra effort is required mentally and physically. When it comes to preparing your daily raw meals, your options are limited. Here are some of the procedures you may apply when organizing your meal plan:

- *Germination* – this is the process of soaking in water for a certain period of time. The recommended amount of time differs from one person to another but for raw foodists, the safest bet is to soak overnight.

- *Sprouting* – this comes after germination. After the beans, legumes or seeds are soaked, they may then be sprouted. Items should be left at room temperature until a sprout comes out of it. These sprouts may then be used for preparing food but should be rinsed and drained thoroughly beforehand.

- *Blending* – involves the use of a blender or food processor in order to create sauces, smoothies, or soup among others.

- *Dehydrating* – employs an equipment known as a dehydrator, which simulates sun drying. Common products of dehydrators are crackers, croutons, raisins, fruit leathers, sundried tomatoes, breads and kale chips.

- *Pickling* – a method of preserving food by marinating in a brine.

- *Juicing* – the process of extracting of vitamins, minerals and natural juices from plant tissues, particularly raw fruits and vegetables.

- *Fermentation* – process of converting sugar to carbon dioxide through the use of yeast.

Now that you know what procedures are available to you when preparing your raw meals, the next thing to know is which particular equipment/s you need to use. Below are some of the staple equipment that can be seen in every raw foodist's kitchen:

- *Dehydrator* – it is an enclosed container that has heating elements that can warm at low temperatures. It has a fan that blows warm air onto the food.

- *Spiral Slicer* – slices vegetables into spiral shapes

- *Thermometer* – to ensure that temperature stays below 118°F when heating food.

- *Trays* – for soaking and sprouting beans, legumes or seeds

- *Sprouters* or *mason jars*

- *Food processor*

- *Blender*

- *Juicer*

These are the basic things you have to know if you intend to convert to the raw food diet. Now that you have an idea of what it is and how it works, you will then have to figure out why you would want to choose this lifestyle.

Chapter 2

Why Do People Go Raw?

To some people, converting to a raw food diet seems like a crazy idea. After all, why would anyone want to give up eating all the delectable cooked dishes for uncooked food? How could one survive solely on salads? Why should you limit your choices when eating? These are just some of the many questions people ask when it comes to changing up their diet. Truth be told, there is a less-than-enthusiastic reception from others. Despite these doubts and uncertainties about the diet, those who choose to go raw are very passionate about adhering to the lifestyle. In fact, raw food diet practitioners more often than not retain this routine for years or even for the rest of their lives.

For those who are wondering why someone would stick to such a challenging and demanding way of life, there are several reasons why people take on the diet. For most, optimal health is the primary objective. Some choose to uphold their philosophical and ethical principles. Then there are others who are merely drawn to the diet's environment-friendly quality. These objectives are further explained below.

Health Reasons

Perhaps the most typical reason why anyone would want to begin a raw food diet is the fact that it is beneficial to one's health. For one, it helps prevent and fight off diseases because of the abundance of vitamins, minerals, nutrients and antioxidants that help reduce risks of illnesses or slow down its progress. It also helps that raw food has a lack of calories, saturated fat, cholesterol and other possibly harmful elements normally found in cooked, processed food. Weight loss is also a huge motivation for raw foodists, since a raw diet rich in fiber and low in calories is a great, fast way to shed pounds. Overall, one's health and well-being is positively affected by the raw food diet.

Philosophical and Ethical Reasons

There are a number of individuals who prefer to apply raw food diet because it is in line with their philosophical and ethical beliefs and principles. These are the same people who refuse to purchase animal meat and processed food. As an alternative, these people choose to support organic agriculture and food coming from plants. A moral code like this is surprisingly a strong incentive for some to go raw.

Environmental Reasons

Environmental benefits were once viewed merely as a bonus as opposed to a primary purpose for going raw, particularly for raw vegan foodists. The cooking and processing of food items also have great effect on the environment. Gigantic amounts of resources are used in the food processing industry. Furthermore, most raw foodists encourage organic agriculture, hence using their money to buy food and advocate against the use of chemical fertilizers, herbicides and pesticides that can damage and eventually destroy the environment.

These are the principal reasons why an individual would want to apply the raw food diet and make it a part of his or her daily routine. Raw foodists have their own opinions and motives for considering such a lifestyle choice.

Chapter 3

Raw Food Recipes to Get You Started

This wide array of recipes will help you sustain a raw food diet without getting tired of eating the same food over and over again.

Sauces, Dressings and Condiments

Most meals are dull and boring without sauces and condiments. A delicious sauce can add more taste and flavor to a dish. However, some worry that by following a diet, one must ultimately give up the use of sauces and condiments. While you cannot use the traditional processed sauces, you may create your own using the recipes below.

1. Silica-Rich Dressing

Cucumbers are packed with the minerals responsible for nourishing connective tissues such as the nails, hair, bones and skin. Moreover, they are naturally refreshing and hydrating. By using cucumbers in this recipe, they allow oil reduction, which makes this dressing a low-calorie option.

Ingredients:

- 1 ¼ cups of cucumber, chopped, peeled and seeded
- 2 tablespoons of apple cider vinegar
- 1 tablespoon of flat-leaf parsley, chopped
- 1 small clove of garlic
- 2 teaspoons of cilantro, chopped
- ¼ cup of extra virgin olive oil
- ¼ teaspoon of dried dill

- ¼ teaspoon of ground black pepper
- ¼ teaspoon of ground red pepper
- ¼ teaspoon of salt

Procedure:

1. Add the cucumber, parsley, cilantro, garlic, vinegar, red pepper, black pepper, dill and salt to a blender or food processor. Blend until smooth.

2. While processing, slowly add the olive oil. Blend for at least 15 seconds or until the oil is fully absorbed.

3. Pour into a container and store in the refrigerator. Shake well before use.

2. Zucchini Hummus

This is similar to the traditional Middle Eastern version but with a highlight on zucchini, which is low on calories. It can be used as a dip, dressing or spread.

Ingredients:

- 1 ½ zucchinis, chopped
- 3 cloves of garlic
- ¾ cup of sesame seeds
- 1/3 cup of parsley, chopped
- 3 ½ tablespoons of lemon juice
- 1/3 teaspoon of salt

Procedure:

1. Blend seeds in a food processor until it achieves a peanut butter-like consistency (tahini). Set aside.

2. Mince the garlic using the food processor.

3. Add the zucchinis, salt, lemon juice and parsley. Process until crudely chopped.

4. Add the tahini to the processor. Blend until smooth.

3. Italian Herb Tomato Sauce

This sauce is easy to prepare and is much healthier. Tomatoes are also rich in several nutrients such as vitamins A and C, folic acid and lycopene. By making the sauce naturally, you get to take advantage of the nutrients that the tomatoes supply. This sauce will go well with other recipes.

Ingredients:

- 2 ½ cups of fresh tomatoes, chopped
- ¼ cup of sun-dried tomatoes
- 2 ½ teaspoon of dried Italian herbs (e.g. oregano, basil, rosemary and parsley)
- 1 clove of garlic
- ½ celery stalk
- 1/3 teaspoon of salt

Procedure:

1. Soak the sun-dried tomatoes preferably overnight or at for at least 2 hours in water until soft.

2. Mince the herbs, salt, garlic and celery in a food processor.

3. Add the soaked sun-dried tomatoes. Blend well and set aside in a large bowl.

4. Place the chopped fresh tomatoes in food processor and process until chunky and saucy.

5. Add to the sun-dried tomato paste. Stir and mix until fully combined.

4. Soured Coconut Cream

Sour cream is a classic dip found in American and European cuisine. This version utilizes coconut to ensure you stick to your diet. It has a tangy taste plus all the healthy nutrients found in coconuts.

Ingredients:

- ¾ cup of fresh young coconut meat
- 2 teaspoons of lemon juice
- ½ teaspoon of onion powder
- ½ teaspoon of garlic powder
- ½ cup of water

Procedure:

1. Using a blender or food processor, blend all the ingredients until smooth and faintly whipped.

2. Place finished product in a lidded glass jar. Refrigerate.

5. Rawbecue Sauce

This is the raw version of the barbecue sauce and can work well either as a marinade, dip or dressing.

Ingredients:

- 1 dried pepper, soaked
- 1 clove of garlic
- 1 cup of sundried tomatoes, soaked
- 1 cup of fresh tomato, chopped
- 2 tablespoons of yacon syrup
- 2 tablespoons of apple cider vinegar
- 2 teaspoons of chili powder
- 1 teaspoon of nama shoyu
- ½ teaspoon of salt
- ½ cup of soaking water

Procedure:

1. In a blender, place all the ingredients together. Blend until smooth.

2. Store the finished sauce in a glass jar with a lid. Refrigerate.

Breakfast

Considered the most important meal of the day, breakfast is the perfect time for raw food enthusiasts to enjoy meals, from fruits and vegetables to classic breakfast meals with a raw twist. A nutritious meal will allow you to retain your energy throughout the day.

1. Walnut Banana Pancakes

Pancakes are a breakfast favorite, and this recipe allows you to enjoy this childhood favorite and still staying true to the raw food diet. Sadly, this is not the kind of pancake that you can make instantly just by mixing.

Ingredients:

- 6 bananas, sliced
- 2 apples, chopped and cored
- 1 ½ cups of buckwheat
- 1 tablespoon of flax seeds
- 1 cup of sunflower seeds
- 2 tablespoons of coconut flakes
- ½ cup of walnuts, chopped
- 1 ¼ tablespoons of ground cinnamon
- ¼ teaspoon of salt

Procedure:

1. Soak the sunflower seeds and buckwheat overnight or for no less than 6 hours. Rinse well before use.

2. In a coffee grinder or blender, process the flax seeds until it turns into powder. Set aside.

17

3. In a food processor, blend sunflower seeds and buckwheat until it gets a creamy consistency. Place in a bowl.

4. Process the bananas, apples, salt and cinnamon until smooth. Add to the bowl.

5. Add the walnuts, coconut flakes and flax seeds to the mixture. Mix thoroughly.

6. Prepare ParaFlexx sheets. Shape pancakes by hand. If you have a dehydrator, dehydrate the mixtures for 8 to 12 hours. Otherwise, use an oven until the mixture is dry on the outside but moist inside.

2. Breakfast Tacos with Ruby Raspberry Filling

The romaine lettuce contains antioxidants in its leaves that is said to help battle cancer. It also helps give this recipe a crunchy feel, which is exactly how tacos should be.

Ingredients:

- Breakfast Tacos with Ruby Raspberry Filling
- The romaine lettuce contains antioxidants in its leaves that is said to help battle cancer. It also helps give this recipe a crunchy feel, which is exactly how tacos should be.
- *Ingredients:*
- 4 to 8 romaine leaves
- 1 ruby red grapefruit
- 1 cup of raspberries
- ½ cup of nectarines, diced
- ½ cup of peaches, diced
- 1 teaspoon to 1 tablespoon of agave syrup (optional)

Procedure:

1. Peel the grapefruit and remove the pith using a sharp knife. Then, slice the fruit in half.

2. Place the grapefruit along with the other ingredients (except the leaves) in a mixing bowl. Add agave and toss.

3. Scoop the mix into the romaine leaves.

3. Killer Kasha Porridge

Kasha is a traditional savory dish popular in numerous countries in Eastern Europe and is usually made from buckwheat. This recipe lets you enjoy this dish in its raw form.

Ingredients:

- 2 cups of buckwheat grouts, soaked and sprouted
- 1 cup of apple, chopped
- 2 teaspoons of orange zest
- 1 tablespoon cinnamon
- ½ teaspoon of sea salt

Procedure:

1. Put all the ingredients in a blender or food processor. Blend until it reaches a porridge-like consistency.

2. Scoop into a bowl and serve.

4. Cinnamon Apple Granola

This enjoyable bowl of crunchy granola is another breakfast favorite. You can change it up and use other fruits such as berries, strawberries or bananas.

Ingredients:

- 2 cups of buckwheat
- 2 apples, cored
- 15 dates, pitted
- ¾ cup of almonds
- ½ cup of cashews
- ¾ cup of Brazil nuts
- 1 ½ cups of sunflower seeds
- ½ cup of pumpkin seeds
- ¾ cup of coconut flakes
- 1 tablespoon of ground cinnamon
- 2 tablespoons of hemp protein powder
- 1 tablespoon of maca powder
- 1 teaspoon of vanilla powder
- ½ teaspoon of salt

Procedure:

1. In a bowl, soak almonds, sunflower seeds, pumpkins and buckwheat overnight. Rinse well before use.

2. In a separate bowl, soak Brazil nuts overnight. Rinse well before use.

3. In another bowl, soak cashews overnight. Rinse well before use.

4. In a food processor, process the Brazil nuts until it achieves a medium fine consistency. Add to the bowl of other seeds and nuts along with the cashews.

5. Add the coconut flakes to the bowl.

6. Process the apples, dates, cinnamon, hemp protein powder, salt, vanilla and maca in the food processor until it gets smooth and saucy. Add to the bowl nuts and seeds. Stir thoroughly by hand.

7. Place layers of the mix on ParaFlexx sheets. Place in a dehydrator at 108°F overnight. If you do not have a dehydrator, use an oven and let it bake until the cashews and almonds are crunchy.

5. Creamy Coconut Yogurt

Yogurt is considered a healing food due to the probiotics it contains which helps colonize the digestive tract. The coconut gives this recipe a creamy backdrop for your fruit or garnish of your choice. Coconuts are also rich in healthy fats, helping you stay full during the day.

Ingredients:

- 2 cups of young Thai coconut meat, shredded
- 1 cup of coconut water
- 1 teaspoon of probiotic powder

Procedure:

1. Place the coconut water and coconut meat in a blender. Blend until creamy.

2. Transfer the mix into a container. Add the probiotic powder and stir.

3. Using a piece of cheesecloth or a towel, cover the container and leave for 4-8 hours to sit at room temperature.

4. Serve in a glass or bowl. Store leftovers in the refrigerator.

Note:

You may choose to add other fruits such as bananas or strawberries to give the yogurt more flavors.

Salads

Being a raw foodist, you probably had someone ask you if salads are all you eat. This is part true; salads are an integral part of the raw food diet and are highly nutritious. But contrary to popular belief, salads are not mundane and flavorless. In fact, here are some delectable salad recipes that you may use.

1. Spiked Citrus Curried Quinoa Salad

Sprouted quinoa is a staple in the raw food diet because it is an amazing source of complete protein. This means it has all the amino acids that the body needs. The addition of the spinach, which provides iron, and the orange juice, which is packed in vitamin C that helps the iron be more absorbable, makes this recipe a very healthy meal.

Ingredients:

- 3 cups of sprouted quinoa
- 4 cups of baby spinach
- 2 scallions, chopped
- ½ cup of orange juice
- 2 tablespoons of olive oil
- 1 teaspoon of curry powder
- ½ teaspoon of coriander powder
- ¾ cup of slivered almonds or pine nuts
- ¾ cup of golden raisins
- ¼ cup of red onion, diced

Procedure:

1. In a large bowl, place the quinoa, onion, raisins and almonds or pine nuts. Toss.

2. In another smaller bowl, whisk the olive oil, orange juice, coriander powder and curry powder together. This will become the dressing of the salad.

3. Drizzle the dressing over the larger bowl of quinoa mixture. Toss completely.

4. Serve the mixture over baby spinach and garnish with scallions.

Notes:

Allow the salad to marinate in the dressing for one hour for better taste.

You may use other dried fruits instead of raisins.

If you want a spicier salad, add sliced jalapeños to the mix.

For a tangier flavor, add tangerine chunks.

2. Lettuce Lover's Salad

If you enjoy greens, then you will love this recipe. This particular recipe emphasizes on lettuce but you can easily change up the recipe and use a different vegetable of your liking such as kale, collards, butter leaf, cabbage, red oak and so much more. After all, variety is the spice of life.

Ingredients:

- 2 cups of romaine lettuce, chopped
- 1 cup of Bibb lettuce, chopped
- ½ cup of red-leaf lettuce, torn
- 1/3 cup of celery, sliced
- ¼ cup of carrots, sliced
- 1 cup of arugula, torn
- 1 cup of endive, torn
- 2 tablespoons of olive oil
- 4 teaspoons of coconut vinegar
- ¼ teaspoon of sea salt
- ¼ teaspoon of agave syrup
- 1/8 teaspoon of onion powder
- 1/8 teaspoon of garlic powder
- 1/8 teaspoon of paprika
- ¼ cup of grape tomatoes, sliced

Procedure:

1. Combine the romaine, Bibb and celery lettuce in a bowl. Add the celery, carrots, arugula and endive. Toss to mix.

2. In a separate bowl, whisk the coconut vinegar, olive oil, agave and all the spices to produce the dressing.

3. Drizzle the dressing over the bowl of salad. Toss thoroughly.

4. Garnish with the grape tomatoes and serve.

3. Sprouted Quinoa, Olive and Tomato Salad

This salad goes well on its own or served with the zucchini hummus on the side.

Ingredients:

- 1 cup of quinoa
- ¼ cup of celery, chopped
- ¼ cup of sun dried tomatoes
- 3/8 cup of sun-dried black olives, pitted
- 2 tablespoons of lime juice
- ¼ teaspoon of salt

Procedure:

1. Soak quinoa for 4 hours. Rinse well before use.

2. Soak the sun-dried tomatoes for 2 hours in water until soft.

3. Dice the tomatoes.

4. Toss all the ingredients in a bowl until thoroughly mixed.

4. Sunset Salad

This colorful salad has a bit of sweetness and a bit of spice and can be enjoyed as an afternoon snack to refuel you. It can also be served with a side of guacamole.

Ingredients:

- 2 cups of romaine lettuce, chopped
- 2 cups of pineapple, cubed
- 1 cup of red-leaf lettuce
- 1 small jalapeño, seeded and minced
- ½ red bell pepper, julienned
- ½ cup of fresh pineapple juice
- 2 tablespoons of apple cider vinegar
- 1 tablespoon of fresh chives, diced
- ¼ teaspoon of sweet paprika
- 1/8 teaspoon of ground black pepper
- 1/8 teaspoon of sea salt

Procedure:

1. In a bowl, place the lettuces, bell pepper and pineapple cubes. Toss to mix.

2. In another smaller bowl, combine the pineapple juice and jalapeño pepper. Add the sea salt, black pepper, paprika and apple cider vinegar to make dressing.

3. Toss the salad with the dressing. Chill the finished product before serving.

4. Garnish with fresh chives and serve.

5. Basic Coleslaw Mix

This is a hydrating coleslaw which you can eat on its own or mix with other dishes. You may also add your own touch to it and add other seasonal vegetables in the recipe.

Ingredients:

- 2 carrots, rinsed and trimmed
- 2 cups of green cabbage, roughly chopped
- 1 ¼ cups of red cabbage, roughly chopped

Procedure:

1. Shred the carrots and both cabbages in a food processor subsequently.

2. Toss all the ingredients in a bowl. Combine well.

Main Courses

The main course is an extremely important part of your daily meal plan. Going on a raw food diet does not necessarily mean that your food choices will be boring and repetitive. In fact, here are some healthy raw food main course recipes that you may easily prepare.

1. Veggie Burger Patties

These patties are not only healthy but are also perfect for people with several food allergies.

Ingredients:

- 3 tablespoons of flax seeds
- 3 to 4 stalks of celery stalks
- 2 carrots, chopped
- ½ cup of onions, chopped
- ½ red bell pepper, chopped
- 1 ½ cups of walnuts
- 3/8 cup of sunflower seeds
- 2 tablespoons of hemp seeds
- 1 tablespoon of protein powder
- 2/3 cup of tomatoes, chopped
- ¾ teaspoon of salt

Procedure:

1. Soak the sunflower seeds and walnuts in water overnight or for at least six hours. Rinse well before use.

2. Using a coffee grinder or blender, grind the flax seeds until powder-like.

31

3. In a food processor, process the tomatoes, carrots, bell peppers, celery, onions, hemp protein and salt into a puree. Place in a bowl.

4. Process the sunflower seeds and walnuts with along with just the right amount of puree to form a paste. Add this to the rest of the puree in the bowl.

5. Add ground flax seeds and hemp seeds. Mix completely by hand.

6. Form the mixture into patties and place on mesh sheets.

7. Let the patties dry using a dehydrator for at least 18 to 24 hours.

2. Petite Beetloaf

This may serve as a main course for two people and the alternative to the usual meat loaf but with healthier, non-meat ingredients. Despite the lack of meat, it contains a hefty dose of protein due to the walnuts and sprouts.

Ingredients:

- ½ cup of cabbage or mung sprouts
- ¼ cup of alfalfa sprouts
- ¼ cup of beets, shredded
- ½ cup of walnuts, soaked for 2 to 4 hours
- 2 tablespoons of celery hearts, chopped
- 2 tablespoons of white or red onion, chopped
- 2 teaspoons of nama shoyu
- Water

Procedure:

1. Using a food processor, grind the walnuts and sprouts along with the nama shoyu.

2. Add the celery, onion and beets to the food processor and process with a bit of water until all the ingredients stick together.

3. Place this mixture in a sheet and shape into a loaf. Dehydrate at 145°F for at least 12 hours.

3. Spiraled Spaghetti Marinara

The marinara is said to be the dish that truly tests the skills of a chef. This version of the famous pasta is perfect for individuals taking on the raw food diet who are lovers of Italian food. In place of the usual flour, zucchini is used to make the noodles.

Ingredients:

- 3 zucchinis
- ½ teaspoon of salt
- ½ cup of soaked sundried tomatoes, soaked water set aside
- 1 cup of tomatoes, chopped
- ½ cup of red bell pepper, chopped
- 1 clove of garlic, minced
- 2 tablespoons of raisins, dates, chopped apples or currants
- 1 tablespoon of olive oil
- 1 ½ teaspoon of any Italian seasoning
- ¼ teaspoon of cayenne pepper powder

Procedure:

1. If you have a spiralizer, use this to turn the zucchinis into long noodles. Otherwise, you may use a vegetable peeler. Stop until you reach the seeds and get rid of the center.

2. Place the zucchini noodles in a bowl and sprinkle the sea salt on top of it. Stir well. Set bowl aside.

3. Using a food processor or blender, process the sundried tomatoes and the water used for soaking together with all the other ingredients except the noodles. Blend until smooth.

4. Gently squeeze the zucchini noodles to completely get rid of any remaining liquid. Mix with the sauce and toss until thoroughly covered. Serve.

34

4. Tahini Pad Thai

Pad Thai is among the most recognizable Thai dishes available and is starting to become a favorite all over the world. This national dish from Thailand dates back years ago. The raw version of the Pad Thai replaces the peanuts with sesame tahini, removes the fish sauce, egg and leaves out the noodles for a fresher, lighter and healthier meal.

Ingredients:

- 3 zucchinis, medium
- 2 carrots, large
- ¼ cup of sundried tomatoes, soaked in water
- ½ cup of soak water
- 1 tablespoon of tahini
- 2 tablespoons of nama shoyu
- 2 tablespoons of lime juice
- 1 tablespoon of agave syrup
- ½ cup of snow peas
- ½ cup of mung bean sprouts
- ¼ cup of scallions, finely sliced
- 1 clove of garlic, minced
- ½ tablespoon of ginger
- 2 to 4 tablespoons of cilantro, minced
- Lime wedges

Procedure:

1. In a blender, place together the tahini, nama shoyu, sundried tomatoes, ginger, lime juice, agave syrup and garlic and blend until smooth. While blending, slowly pour in the soak water until the mixture turns thick. This will become your pad thai sauce.

2. Turn the carrots and zucchini into noodles using a spiralizer, mandolin or a peeler. You may choose to grate or julienne them alternatively.

3. On a plate, place your noodles, scallions, snow peas and mung bean sprouts. Add the sauce and garnish with the cilantro and lime wedges.

5. Juicy Hues Stir-Dry

This is a vibrant meal, both for the eyes and the mouth, due to the bright colors of the ingredients and their various strong flavors. This main course has the right amount of saltiness, spice and sweetness that you will surely love.

Ingredients:

- 2 cloves of garlic
- 1 red bell pepper, chopped
- 1 orange or yellow bell pepper, chopped
- 1 mango, cubed
- 1 bunch of broccoli, chopped
- 3 scallions, chopped
- 3 tablespoons of nama shoyu
- 2 tablespoons of orange juice
- 1 tablespoon of lime juice
- 1 tablespoon of olive oil
- 1 tablespoon of hot sauce

Procedure:

1. Whisk together the garlic, nama shoyu, lime juice, orange juice, olive oil and hot sauce in a small bowl. Set aside.

2. In a bigger bowl for mixing, toss the mango, bell peppers and broccoli together. Pour the prepared dressing onto the bowl and thoroughly mix until well-coated.

3. Cover the bowl and let it marinate overnight in the refrigerator or for at least 2 hours at room temperature.

4. After letting it marinate, place the bowl to a dehydrator at 110°F for another 2 hours.

5. Garnish using the scallions and serve.

Conclusion

Thank you again for purchasing this book!

I hope this book was able to help you to get a better idea of the raw food diet and provide you with a vast selection of recipes to assure variety in your diet plan.

Change can be overwhelming at times, especially when you are just about to start out. However, if you do not make the changes that are necessary to make your life better, then you will only continue to hold yourself back. If you want to make improvements to your health and whole well-being, the raw food diet may just be the solution you need.

With the raw food diet, you need not rush into anything. You may take things slow and tinker with your routines until you find the right setup for you. While it may be challenging, the rewards that you will reap will all be worth the sacrifice. Let this book be your starting point in progressing towards a raw and healthy lifestyle.

Finally, if you enjoyed this book, please take the time to share your thoughts and post a positive review on Amazon. It'd be greatly appreciated!

In addition, please remember to check out our Facebook page in order to find other resources and upcoming promotions:

https://www.facebook.com/joypublishing

With sincere thanks,

Emma Rose

Preview of 'Clean Eating Guide'
Lose Weight Quickly, Achieve Optimal Health and Feel Energized with Clean Eating for Busy Families and Clean Eating Recipes

Chapter 1
What is Clean Eating?

You have probably come across the term 'clean eating' but you are still not familiar about its exact meaning. This is being used by people who work in the health and fitness industry such as personal trainers ad dietitians. People who are health conscious and workout fanatic also often use this word. Does it have something to do with cleaning the food before eating or cooking? Or maybe it has something to do with the kind of food that you eat.

The loose definition of clean eating is eating food in its most natural state. These days, people are starting to pay more attention to the kinds of food that they eat and how these foods are made. They take note of the food's ingredients and make sure that the food product only contains all natural ingredients.

The term clean eating first came out in the 1990s. Today, it is still being used by health conscious individuals from different backgrounds and culture to refer to the kind of all natural diet that they have. The definition of clean eating can vary from person to person. Some define clean eating as eating mostly fruits and vegetables while others define it as not eating anything artificial. You will find out more about these things as you read this book.

What Clean Eating is not?

If you think clean eating is another diet program, like the South Beach diet or Paleo diet, you are wrong because clean eating is a way of life. It also does not follow any strict rules about what food group to eat and not to eat, how many calories you should consume in a meal, and so on. This is the most basic way of healthy eating that promotes weight loss and boost energy. Everybody can do this, even those who are not trying to lose weight.

Clean eating will not make you feel deprived or frustrated because it is so easy to follow. You do not even need to have a really strong determination because it is all a matter of choosing natural over artificial.

Is there such a thing as 'dirty' eating?

You are probably wondering if there is such a thing as 'dirty' eating or the opposite of clean eating. Clean eating does not literally mean eating foods that have less dirt. It means that you are choosing the best and healthiest food choices from different food groups in their most natural state. 'Dirty' eating is not the opposite of clean eating because there is no such thing as eating dirty. The opposite of clean eating is choosing the wrong food to eat and eating junk foods and processed foods that leave toxins in your body.

Clean eating also looks at the source of food. It should not come from large commercial manufacturers that use machines to process food. The foods that clean eaters usually use come from small farms that do not use chemicals and undergo processes. This is why clean eating is often associated with organic eating.

Check *out the rest of 'Clean Eating Guide' on Amazon*

Or go to: http://amzn.to/UVzNER

Check Out My Other Books

Below you'll find some of my other books also available on Amazon and Kindle. Search for these titles on the Amazon website to find them.

Paleo Free Diet Guide for Beginners: Over 50 Paleo Free Recipes for Optimal Health & Fast Weight Loss

Paleo Desserts: Satisfy Your Sweet Tooth With Over 100 Quick & Easy Paleo Dessert Recipes & Paleo Baking Recipes

Raw Food Diet Guide: Lose Weight Quickly, Achieve Optimal Health & Feel Energized with the Raw Food Diet & Raw Food Recipes

Clean Eating Guide: Lose Weight Quickly, Achieve Optimal Health & Feel Energized with Clean Eating For Busy Families & Clean Eating Recipes

Alkaline Diet Guide: Lose Weight Quickly, Achieve Optimal Health & Feel Energized with the Alkaline Diet & Alkaline Recipes

Coconut Flour Recipes for Optimal Health & Quick Weight Loss: Gluten Free Recipes for Celiac Disease, Gluten Sensitivities & Paleo Free Diets

Almond Flour Recipes for Optimal Health & Quick Weight Loss: Gluten Free Recipes for Celiac Disease, Gluten Sensitivities & Paleo Free Diets

Wheat Free Diet for Beginners: Lose Weight Quickly, Achieve Optimal Health & Feel Energized with Gluten Free Recipes for Celiac Disease, Gluten Sensitivities & Paleo Free Diets

Detox Diet Guide: Lose Weight Quickly, Achieve Optimal Health & Feel Energized Through the 10 Day Detox

Sugar Detox Guide for Beginners: Lose Weight Quickly, Achieve Optimal Health, Feel Energized & Eliminate Sugar Cravings Naturally

Ketogenic Diet Guide for Beginners: How to Achieve Rapid Weight Loss, Optimal Health & Unstoppable Energy with Ketogenic Diet Recipes

Anti Inflammatory Diet for Beginners: Lose Weight Fast, Optimize Health, Slow Aging, Fight Inflammation, Conquer Pain & Increase Energy with the Anti Inflammation Diet Recipes

One Last Thing...

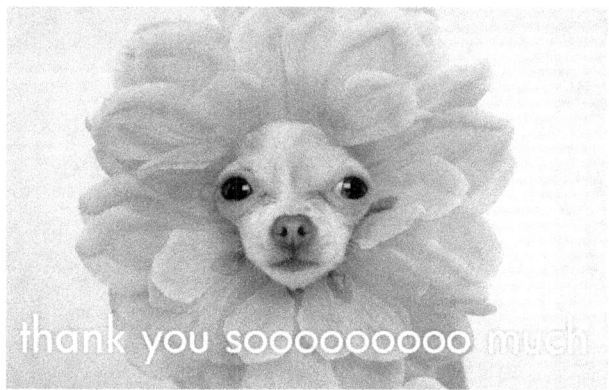

If you believe that this book is worth sharing, would you please take the time to let others know how it affected your life? If it turns out to make a difference in the lives of others, they will be forever grateful to you, as will I.